Smoothies:

Healthy Green Smoothie 30 Day Plan to Lose Weight, Detoxify, Fight Disease, and Live Long

Table of Contents

Introduction

Congratulations on downloading *Smoothies: Healthy Green Smoothie 30 Day Plan to Lose Weight, Detoxify, Fight Disease, and Live Long* and thank you for doing so. When it comes to improving your overall quality of life, there are few better things you can do for your body than purify it of all the unhealthy toxins that build up naturally over the years and making the decision to take charge of your diet and improve yourself is a decision worth celebrating.

Unfortunately deciding to make a positive change in your diet is much easier than actually going through with what needs to be done in order to do so which is why the following chapters will discuss everything you need in order to get started on your new lifestyle and stick with it in the long term. First you will learn all about the many benefits that green smoothies can have when it comes to detoxifying your system and helping you lose weight as quickly and easily as possible. From there, you will then be provided with an outline of a meal plan that will further compound the process and make it easier for you to succeed. Finally, you will be provided with 60 different green smoothie recipes to ensure that you can find the smoothie (or smoothies) that are right for you.

There are plenty of books on this subject on the market, thanks again for choosing this one! Every effort was made to ensure it is full of as much useful information as possible, please enjoy!

Chapter 1: Green Smoothie Basics

When it comes to easily getting all the nutrients that you need for the day while at the same time losing weight and detoxifying your system, there are few better options available than a green smoothie. While the idea of the green smoothie is relatively straight forward, any smoothie that is composed of at least 70 percent leafy, dark greens can be said to be green, the space is vast enough that it can be confusing for those just starting out to know where to begin. While the specifics might vary, all green smoothies are sure to share a variety of health benefits, regardless of the specific fruits and vegetables that you choose to use.

Easily digestible
Studies have proven that vegetables and fruits that have been blended together are naturally healthier than if those same vegetables and fruits were consumed in their natural state. While this might seem counterintuitive, the blending process breaks down the cell walls present in the cells of all plants, making it easier for your body to extract the required nutrients in the process. In a nutshell, the blending process acts as the initial stages of digestion leaving your body free to expend its energy on absorbing as much nutrition from the things that you put into it as possible. As an added bonus, the fiber found in green smoothies also improves digestion overall by forcing your colon to work overtime.

Brimming with nutrition

With 70 percent of every smoothie being made up of healthy greens, it stands to reason that each smoothie you consume is going to run the gamut when it comes to vitamins and minerals. They are also known to contain a dramatically higher concentration of antioxidants and polyphenols which are extremely important when it comes to fighting off degenerative diseases, including cancer. Pound for pound, when compared to juices made from the same raw materials, smoothies contain nearly five times as much fiber as well.

Great replacement for caffeine

While caffeine is a great way to get an extra burst of energy in a short period of time, it is largely void of any real nutritional value. Compare this with the average green smoothie which is so full of vitamins and nutrients that the energy it provides is enough to give a jolt to the system practically on par with a cup of coffee. This makes green smoothies a great way to start the day or to get you through the midafternoon doldrums in style.

Excellent way to detoxify your system

When it comes to initiating a 30-day detox, green smoothies are a natural choice for flushing your system of a wide variety of toxins. They are so effective thanks to the high amount of chlorophyll that they contain which naturally encourages the cells in the human body to release toxins that they have been holding onto for years, if not decades. The previously mentioned high amounts of fiber also stimulate the colon to ensure it is active for its part of the detoxification process as well.

What's more, it doesn't take a massive amount of green smoothie consumption to begin seeing these benefits either, nor does it require a radical restructuring of your diet beyond simply making a concentrated effort to eat healthy and avoid foods that are naturally high in toxins. For most people two servings of a green smoothie per day is enough to start seeing real results if they keep it up for just a few weeks.

Easy to make and very portable
One of the biggest reasons that many people find themselves unable to maintain a healthy diet is that it can be difficult to find healthy foods on the go. The green smoothie takes care of these concerns as practically all green smoothies can be ready to go in less than 5 minutes and each preparation can easily make 2 or more servings. As long as there is a cool place for storage, most of the smoothies in the following pages will keep for about 24 hours meaning that 5 minutes in the morning is all you need to set yourself up for success for the entire day.

Something for everyone
The 70/30 split for a proper green smoothie means that they are sure to be palatable both for dedicated vegetarians as well as those who believe that vegetables are strictly only what real food eats. Thirty percent fruit is enough to cut the flavors of many of the healthiest vegetable to a point that you won't even know they

are there. While it might take you a few days to adapt to the taste, your pallet will typically adapt within as little as 7 days and you will be surprised how quickly you start to crave a healthy alternative to sugary snacks or a quick fast food meal that is completely devoid of all nutritional content.

Chapter 2: Tips and Tricks for Success

Choose the right blender for the job

For those just getting into the smoothie game, the wide variety of potential tools can make it difficult to separate the wheat from the chaff. First and foremost, it is important to look for a powerful blender instead of a juicer. A juicer extracts the essence of fruits and vegetables, leaving all of the healthy pulp and all of its related nutrients behind. Rather, you are going to want to invest in a blender, and a quality one at that, in order to make your green smoothie transition as easy as possible.

When it comes to choosing a blender the first thing that you are going to want to consider is the quality of the motor to ensure that it will be able to stand up to all of the stress of daily blending that you will be subjecting it too. While they are going to be more expensive, it is recommended that you choose a blender that is 1000 watts or more which will ensure that it is able to fully liquify anything that crosses its path. To ensure that it lives up to your standards, you should also make sure it has a warranty that is good for a year, if not longer. Finally, you want to ensure that it has a nice wide mouth and enough room to hold about 40 ounces of liquid if you don't want to have to blend multiple times each day.

If you already have a blender that you feel is mostly adequate to the task at hand, and you don't relish spending approximately

$400 on the type of blender that makes smoothie making as easy as possible, there are a number of things you can do to ensure that your smoothies turn out as smooth as possible. First you are going to want to ensure that you always add any liquid ingredients first as this will create more suction in your blender which will pull any other ingredients you add more fully into the blades. Depending on the strength of your blender, as much as 16 ounces of liquid might be required.

Next, if the smoothie that you are making contains fruit, it is important to add it in before you start in on the greens. This only goes for fresh fruit, however, as frozen fruit should only be added after any fresh ingredients but before any extra ice you may be inclined to add. Adding the fruit before the vegetables will help to ensure that there is enough suction to get the vegetables right down next to the blades where they can do the most good.

When it comes to vegetables, you are going to want to pre-chop, shred or dice your ingredients based on the strength of your blender's motor. If you have a standard 300-watt motor you will want to avoid adding anything that has a diameter greater than 1 inch with weaker motors requiring even smaller pieces. This is one of the most compelling to go with either a Blendtec or Vitamix blender as their stronger motors will save you a significant amount of time in the long run.

To reach the right blending consistency, you are going to want to vary the speed on your blender while also making judicious use of the pulse button. Pulsing at the start will like break up many of the more hearty parts of your smoothie and make the rest of the blending process much easier as a result. Once you have started things moving with the pulse button, you will then want to slowly work your way up the speeds at your disposal, increasing the speed approximately every 30 seconds. If you have to stop in the middle of the process for any reason it is recommended that you start off at the slowest speed when you resume and repeat the process.

If your smoothies end up being more of a food that you chew rather than a liquid that you drink, you may find it effective to pulse for up to two minutes prior to starting the alternating speed process. If you still aren't getting the results that you would like you may need to start with any liquids or berries that you are using and blending them completely before adding in your greens in two or more phases, slowly working up to the tougher vegetables. Even with an underpowered blender you should be able to ultimately create an acceptable smoothie, it will just take much longer and be a more elaborate process than something with the power to get it all done at once.

Take it slow
If the smoothies that you end up with are still a little on the chewy side, it is important to pace yourself during consumption to give your body the opportunity to digest all of the plant

11

matter that you are suddenly consuming. While this is not an issue if your smoothie doesn't require any chewing, if you do find yourself masticating more than you would like then the enzymes in your stomach are likely working overtime and overloading them is a great way to give yourself a stomachache.

The same thing can occur with non-organic fruit and vegetables of the sort that are commonly found in traditional grocery stores. While organic fruits and vegetables are recommended as they typically are more nutritious and contain fewer chemicals and pesticides, using more traditional produce is acceptable as long as you scrub each ingredient thoroughly to ensure you are avoiding consuming a large amount of potential dangerous chemicals. The most reliable way to ensure your fruits and vegetables are chemical and pesticide free is to soak them for anywhere from 15 to 20 minutes in a mixture of water combined with .5 cups of apple cider vinegar and then rinsing each off individually.

Add variety to your diet
When you are first starting out with green smoothies, it can be easy to find a few different recipes that you like and stick with them to the exclusion of everything else. While understandable, this mindset deprives you of one of the greatest strengths of the green smoothie, the variety that is inherent in the fruits and vegetables that become available with the changing of the seasons. Different fruits and vegetables have different levels of many different vitamins and nutrients and following the

changing of the seasons is a quick and easy way to ensure that you are getting a well-round and varied diet. What's more, mixing things up gives you an opportunity to find new favorites that you never would have discovered otherwise.

Chapter 3: 30 Day Plan Explained

The following chapters contain 7 days worth of meals, breakfasts, lunches, dinners and desserts, chosen with the aim to help you detox your system as effectively as possible while at the same time helping you to lose weight along the way. In addition to following the suggested meal plan you should plan on drinking one or two of the smoothies listed in chapter 11 to kick your 30-day detox into high gear. Once you have tried the meals in the order in which they are listed, from there you are free to mix and match for the remainder of the 30 days to create a meal plan that is unique for you. Below is the shopping list for the first 7 days.

<u>Vegetables</u>

- Avocado (5)
- Red cabbage (1)
- Chili (1)
- Carrots (15)
- Yellow pepper (1)
- Edamame (1.5 c)
- Spearmint leaves (12)
- Cucumber (1)
- Garlic (16 cloves)
- Broccoli (4 heads)
- Red bell pepper (9)

- Scallions (19)
- Sun dried tomatoes (1 T)
- Spinach (32 oz)
- Kale (1 c)
- Mushrooms (.25 c)
- Basil (1.5 c)
- Pepperoncino peppers (2)
- Tomatoes (5, 2 lb canned)
- Tomato pesto (.25 c)
- Butternut squash (2)
- Celery (3 stalks)
- Yellow Onion (1)
- Vegetable broth (8 c)
- Onion (5)
- Chives (1 bunch)
- Green Beans (1 lb)
- Orange Pepper (1)
- Yellow pepper (1)
- Cauliflower (1 head)
- Corn kernels (3.5 c)
- Cilantro (1 c)
- Cherry Tomatoes (1 c)
- English cucumber (1)
- Green onion (6)
- Baby potatoes (2 lbs)
- Peas (1 cup frozen)

- Black olive tapenade (.75 c)
- Sweet potato (1)
- Sunflower sprouts (1 handful)

Grains

- Quinoa (4.25 c)
- Corn tortilla 6 inch (8)
- Wheat tortilla 7 inch (1)
- Wheat spaghetti (1 lb)
- English muffin (3)
- Whole grain crackers (5)
- Rice noodles (1 lb)
- Steel cut oats (.25 c)
- Rolled oats (1.25 c)
- Rice (1 c)
- Barley (.25 c)
- Farro (.3 c)

Meat

- Chicken breast (2.5 lb)
- Shrimp (1.5 lbs)
- Smoked Salmon (2 oz)

Beans

- White beans (1 can)
- Red lentils (1 can)
- Kidney beans (1 can)
- Black beans (1 can)
- Garbanzo beans (1 can)
- Baked beans (1 can)

Eggs/Dairy

- Egg (24)
- Buttermilk (1 c)
- Plain Greek Yogurt (5 c)
- Sour cream (.25 c)
- Feta Cheese (2 T)
- Vanilla yogurt fat free (24 oz)
- Pecorino Romano cheese (2 T)
- Milk (4 c)
- Paneer (16 oz)
- Soy milk (2.5 c)
- Cheddar cheese (1 oz)
- Mozzarella cheese (16 oz)
- Lemon yogurt (6 oz)

Seasonings/Sweeteners

- Ketchup (2 T)
- Honey (1.25 c)

- Cinnamon (1.75 tsp ground)
- Vanilla extract (2 tsp)
- Ginger (7 inches)
- Rice vinegar (1 c)
- Red pepper flakes (2 T)
- Arrowroot powder (6.5 tsp)
- Soy sauce (1 c)
- Hot sauce (6 oz)
- Salsa (4 T)
- Chicken bone broth (.5 c)
- Cumin (2.5 tsp)
- Vanilla (1 tsp)
- Black pepper (4 T)
- Lime juice (1 T)
- Lemon juice (1 tsp)
- Nutmeg (.75 tsp)
- Peanut butter (.5 c)
- Cardamom (.5 tsp)
- Cloves (3)
- Paprika (3 T)
- Coriander (.5 c)
- Turmeric (1 T)
- Red chili powder (1 tsp)
- Miso (2 T)
- Gingersnap (1)
- Chocolate chips (.25 c)

- Taco seasoning (1 T)
- Maple syrup (3 T)
- Cayenne pepper (2.25 tsp)
- Garam masala (2 tsp)
- Tarragon (.5 tsp)
- Parsley (2 T)
- Mayonnaise (.25 c)

Fruits

- Raspberries (1.5 c)
- Blueberries (2 c)
- Lemon (1)
- Crushed pineapple (1.5 c)
- Cranberries (1 cups)
- Apple Juice (.5 c)
- Goji Berries (.25 c)

Oils/Butter

- Canola oil (3 c)
- Margarine (3 T)
- Sesame Oil (4 T)
- Olive oil (16 T)
- Extra virgin olive oil (4 T)
- Flaxseed oil (4 T)
- Coconut oil (1 T)

Nuts/Seeds

- Walnuts (1 c chopped)
- Sesame seeds (1 T)
- Chia seeds (.5 oz)
- Flax seeds (.5 oz)
- Pomegranate seeds (.5 oz)
- Fenugreek seeds (1 T)
- Almond milk (.3 c)
- Pecans (1.25 c)
- Cashews (.3 c)
- Almonds (2 c)

Baking

- Celtic salt (10 tsp)
- Sea salt (2 tsp)
- Baking soda (2.5 tsp)
- Baking powder (17 T)
- Sugar (2 c)
- Yellow cornmeal (2 c)
- Whole wheat flour (5.25 c)
- All-purpose flour (4.25 c)
- Pancake mix (1.5 c)
- Brown sugar (4 T)

Chapter 4: Day 1

Breakfast: Fruity, Nutty Pancakes

For this recipe, you will need to set aside 10 minutes for preparation, 20 minutes of cooking time and the results will feed 4.

Nutrition Information

255 calories

10 g of protein

387 mg of sodium

5 g of fiber

2 g of fat (saturated)

67 g of carbs

15 g of fat

Ingredients-Pancake Batter

- Whole wheat flour (1.5 c)

- Sugar (6 T)

- Salt (.5 tsp)

- Baking powder (1 T)

- Flour (1.5 c)

- Baking soda (1 tsp)

Ingredients-Pancakes

- Buttermilk (1 c)

- Egg (1)

- Water (.25 c)
- Cinnamon (.25 tsp)
- Banana (1 thinly sliced)
- Canola oil (1 T)
- Pancake mix (1.3 c)
- Raspberries (.5 c)
- Vanilla extract (1 tsp)
- Honey (.3 c)
- Water (1 T)
- Walnuts (.5 c chopped)

Cooking instructions

- Place the cornmeal, both types of flour, baking powder, sugar, baking soda and salt into a mixing bowl and combine thoroughly.
- Take 1.3 c of the results and mix with the cinnamon in a separate bowl.
- In yet another bowl, combine the buttermilk, egg, water, vanilla extract and canola oil and mix thoroughly before adding in the banana slices.
- In a final bowl, combine the walnuts, honey and 1 T water.
- Prepare a skillet before setting it on the stove above a burner set to medium.
- .25 c of batter will make one pancake. Each side of each pancake will need to cook for approximately 2 minutes.

- Top the finished pancakes using the honey mixture and the raspberries.

Lunch: Sesame and Ginger Quinoa Salad

For this recipe, you will need to set aside 10 minutes for preparation, 15 minutes of cooking time and the results will feed 4.

Nutrition Information
363 calories
15 g of protein
197 mg of sodium
8 g of fiber
2 g of fat (saturated)
43 g of carbs
14 g of fat

Ingredients
- Water (2 c)
- Edamame (1.5 c)
- Quinoa (1 c rinsed)
- Salt (.25 tsp)
- Carrots (3 medium diced)
- Chili (.5 diced)
- Yellow pepper (.5 diced)
- Sesame oil (2 T)
- Rice vinegar (2 T)

- Red cabbage (1 c chopped)
- Sesame seeds (1 T)
- Ginger (.4 tsp)

<u>Cooking instructions</u>
- Turn a boiler to a high heat before combining the water, quinoa and salt together in a covered pot and placing the pot on the boiler. After it reaches the boiling point reduce the heat to low and let the quinoa cook 15 minutes or until the water is completely absorbed.
- Combine the peppers, carrots, cabbage, edamame and the quinoa in a bowl and mix well.
- Separately in another bowl, combine the ginger, sesame oil, rice vinegar and sesame seeds together and mix well.
- Combine the two bowls prior to serving.

Dinner: Garlic Chicken with Soy Sauce and Ginger

For this recipe, you will need to set aside 20 minutes for preparation, 12 minutes of cooking time and the results will feed 4.

Nutrition Information
394 calories
51 g of protein
1120 mg of sodium
2.8 g of fiber
1 g of fat (saturated)

25 g of carbs

10.4 g of fat

Ingredients

- Soy sauce (.5 c)
- Arrowroot powder (3.5 tsp)
- Ginger (2 T chopped)
- Water (.5 c)
- Honey (.25 c)
- Broccoli (16 oz)
- Garlic (2 cloves)
- Chicken breast (2 lbs)
- Olive oil (2 T)
- Carrots (4 sliced)
- Red pepper flakes (as needed)

Cooking instructions

- In a small bowl, mixt together the arrowroot powder, water, honey and soy sauce.
- Place the results into a sauce pan before setting the pan above a burner to a medium/low. Allow the sauce 5 minutes to thicken, stir approximately once per minute.
- Set a large skillet above a burner turned to medium/high and coat it with the olive oil. Add in the chicken as well as the carrots stirring regularly and let it cook approximately 7 minutes before adding in the garlic and cooking another minute.

- While waiting for the chicken to cook, microwave the broccoli until it is cooked to your desired level of firmness.
- Once the broccoli has cooked, add the sauce to the skillet and mix well.
- Top with red pepper flakes as desired before serving.

Dessert: Banana Bread with Blueberries

For this recipe, you will need to set aside 10 minutes for preparation, 40 minutes of cooking time and the results will feed 16.

Nutrition Information
197 calories
5 g of protein
134 mg of sodium
2 g of fiber
1 g of fat (saturated)
29 g of carbs
8 g of fat

Ingredients
- Baking soda (.5 tsp)
- Banana (3)
- Avocado (.25 c)
- Sugar (.75 c)
- Baking soda (.5 tsp)

- Salt (1 tsp)
- Whole wheat flour (.5 c)
- Baking powder (1 tsp)
- Whole wheat flour (.5 c)
- Vanilla extract (1 tsp)
- Eggs (3)
- Blueberries (.5 c)
- Water (3 T)
- Margarine (3 T)

Cooking instructions

- Set your oven to 350 degrees F beforehand
- Combine the baking soda and the bananas in a mixing bowl.
- In another bowl, combine the avocado, sugar and margarine before then adding in the eggs one by one. Next, add in the salt, baking powder, all of the flour and mix enough for the ingredients to begin to combine.
- Combine the two bowls before adding in the water and vanilla, finally fold in the blueberries.
- Add the results to two 8 in loaf pans and let them bake for 40 minutes. The bread is finished when an inserted toothpick comes out clean.
- Cool 5 minutes prior to serving.

Chapter 5: Day 2

Breakfast: Huevoes Rancheros with a Spicy Kick

For this recipe, you will need to set aside 10 minutes for preparation, 16 minutes of cooking time and the results will feed 4.

Nutrition Information

331 calories

16 g of protein

245 mg of sodium

10 g of fiber

3 g of fat (saturated)

42 g of carbs

12 g of fat

Ingredients

- White beans (16 oz)
- Red bell pepper (1 stripped)
- Cumin (1 tsp)
- Scallions (4 sliced)
- Garlic (2 minced cloves)
- Chicken broth (.5 c)
- Plain Greek Yoghurt (4 T)
- Avocado (1 c peeled, sliced)
- Eggs (4)
- Hot sauce (as needed)

- Salsa (4 T)
- Six-inch corn tortillas (8)

Cooking instructions

- Apply cooking spray to your skillet before placing it on the stove above a burner set to a medium/high heat.
- Add the cumin to the skillet and allow it 30 seconds to cook, stirring continuously. Once it becomes fragrant, mix in the red bell pepper, chicken broth, scallions, garlic and beans.
- Allow the ingredients in the skillet to boil before turning the heat down and letting everything simmer for 8 minutes until the skillet is nearly devoid of broth. Once this occurs mash the beans until the results are lumpy.
- Create 4 separate indentations in the beans before cracking the eggs and adding one to each indentation.
- Place a lid on your skillet and let the eggs cook until they reach the state which you prefer.
- Split the results in the skillet into 4 before topping with the avocado, salsa, yoghurt and hot sauce. Serve with tortillas.

Lunch: Kale and Spinach Feta Wrap

For this recipe, you will need to set aside 10 minutes for preparation, 6 minutes of cooking time and the results will feed 1.

Nutrition Information

252 calories

16.2 g of protein

600 mg of sodium

5 g of fiber

4.5 g of fat (saturated)

23 g of carbs

11 g of fat

Ingredients

- Mushrooms (.25 c sliced)
- Spinach (1 c)
- Feta cheese (2 T)
- Whole wheat tortilla (7 in)
- Black pepper (.25 tsp)
- Kale (1 c)
- Sun dried tomatoes (1 T chopped)
- Egg (1)
- Egg white (1 whisked)

Cooking instructions

- Warm the tortilla by placing it in the microwave and letting it cook for 1 minute on the standard power setting.
- At the same time, coat a skillet using cooking spray before placing it on the stop above a burner turned to a medium heat. Place the mushrooms into the skillet before

seasoning with the pepper and letting them cook for 2 minutes.

- Mix in the spinach and let it cook until it begins to wilt which should take approximately another 2 minutes.
- Mix in the egg and let them cook until they have begun to set which should take approximately 2 more minutes.
- Place the results into the tortilla and top with the feta cheese and chopped sun dried tomato prior to serving.

Dinner: Pasta Topped with Spinach and Homemade Tomato Sauce

For this recipe, you will need to set aside 25 minutes for preparation, 12 minutes of cooking time and the results will feed 4.

Nutrition Information
399 calories
14.5 g of protein
818 mg of sodium
9 g of fiber
4 g of fat (saturated)
41 g of carbs
15.5 g of fat

Ingredients

- Whole wheat spaghetti (1 lb)
- Garlic (4 cloves chopped)

- Fresh spinach (10 oz)
- Pecorino Romano cheese (2 T)
- Tomatoes (4 chopped)
- Dried pepperoncino peppers (2 chopped)
- Sea salt (1 tsp)
- Basil (.5 c chopped)
- Extra virgin olive oil (2.5 T)

Cooking instructions

- Place the pasta into a medium-sized pot and let it cook according to the provided directions
- While the pasta is cooking, place your skillet onto the stove above a burner turned to a medium heat. Coat the skillet using the olive oil before adding in the pepperoncino peppers and letting them cook for 60 seconds before mixing in the garlic and letting the results cook until the garlic begins to smell fragrant but has not yet burned.
- Mix in the tomatoes and let them cook for 10 minutes or until they are fully cooked and a little soft, stir regularly. Top with the cheese and add in the salt before pouring the results into an immersion blender to thoroughly combine the ingredients.
- Add the results back into the skillet and then add in the basil, spinach and pasta.
- Combine well prior to serving.

Dessert: Carrot Cake Muffins

For this recipe, you will need to set aside 10 minutes for preparation, 25 minutes of cooking time and the results will feed 12.

Nutrition Information
209 calories
9 g of protein
226 mg of sodium
1 g of fiber
2 g of fat (saturated)
32 g of carbs
6 g of fat

Ingredients

- Flour (1.25 c)
- Salt (.25 tsp)
- Whole wheat flour (.5 c)
- Cinnamon (1 tsp)
- Baking soda (.25 tsp)
- Baking powder (1 tsp)
- Sour cream (.25 c)
- Cream cheese (.5 c)
- Canola oil (2 T)
- Sugar (2.5 T)
- Vanilla (1 tsp)
- Brown sugar (2.5 T)

- Egg (1)
- Carrots (1 c)
- Pineapple (.5 c crushed)

Cooking instructions

- Set your oven ahead of time to 375 degrees F
- Place muffin cups into a 12-slot muffin tin
- In a small mixing bowl combine the sugar, cream cheese and egg together and mix well before adding in the pineapple as well as the carrots
- In a separate bowl, mix together the sour cream, canola oil, sugar and brown sugar and blend well before mixing in the vanilla.
- Ensure there is space in the dry ingredients for the wet ingredients before coming the two bowls and mixing well. Take care not to overmix.
- Fill the muffin tins with the results, taking care to leave room in each space for the baked muffin to rise.
- Add the tin to the preheated oven and bake for 20 minutes. The muffins will be fully cooked when you can stick a toothpick into the center of the center muffins and it comes out clean.
- Allow the muffins 20 minutes to cool before serving.

Chapter 6: Day 3

Breakfast: Tomato Pesto and Eggs Florentine

For this recipe, you will need to set aside 25 minutes for preparation, 5 minutes of cooking time and the results will feed 4.

Nutrition Information
175 calories
12 g of protein
462 mg of sodium
5 g of fiber
2 g of fat (saturated)
21 g of carbs
6 g of fat

Ingredients
- Spinach (10 oz)
- Plain Greek yoghurt (.5 c)
- Olive oil (1 tsp)
- Vinegar (1 tsp)
- Sun dried tomato pesto (.25 cups)
- Eggs (4 large)
- Black pepper (as needed)
- Salt (1 pinch)
- English muffin (2 toasted)

<u>Cooking instructions</u>

- Use the olive oil to prepare the skillet before adding it to the stove above a burner set to a medium/high heat.

- Add in the spinach and let it cook for approximately 2 minutes until it begins to wilt. Once this happens, add in the tomato pesto along with the Greek yoghurt and mix well. Remove the skillet from the stove.

- Pour 1 in of water into a saucepan before placing the pan on the stove above a burner that is set to a high heat. Let the water boil and then add in the vinegar along with the salt before turning the heat to low.

- Place one of the eggs into a cup and then add it gently to the water, repeating the process with the remaining eggs. Place a lid on the skillet and allow the eggs to simmer for about 5 minutes, shaking the pan once every 1.5 minutes.

- Split the English muffins in two before placing each on a plate before toping it with some of the spinach. Use a slotted spoon to top each muffin with an egg.

- Add what is left into the skillet before combining it with the pesto and yogurt and mix thoroughly prior to topping each muffin with the results.

Lunch: Butternut Squash and Lentil Soup

For this recipe, you will need to set aside 5 minutes for preparation, 8 hours of cooking time and the results will feed 8.

Nutrition Information
253 calories

18.3 g of protein

792 mg of sodium

17 g of fiber

0 g of fat (saturated)

41 g of carbs

2 g of fat

Ingredients

- Vegetable broth (8 c)
- Red lentils (2 c)
- Nutmeg (.5 tsp)
- Yellow onion (1 chopped)
- Carrots (3 sliced)
- Butternut squash (3 c diced)
- Garlic (2 cloves minced)

Cooking instructions

- In a slow cooker, add the yellow onion, butternut squash, vegetable broth, red lentils, carrots, garlic and celery.
- Place a lid on the slow cooker before turning it to a low heat and letting it cook for 8 hours. You can also cook the soup for 5 hours if you use a high heat instead.
- The resulting soup can be successfully stored in the refrigerator for approximately 3 days, after that it should be moved to the freezer.

Dinner: Tikka Masala

For this recipe, you will need to set aside 45 minutes for preparation, 20 minutes of cooking time and the results will feed 6.

Nutrition Information

525 calories

19 g of protein

700 mg of sodium

0 g of fiber

1.5 g of fat (saturated)

28 g of carbs

15 g of fat

Ingredients-Gravy

- Sea salt (1 tsp)
- Canned tomatoes (1 lb, chopped)
- Olive oil (3 T)
- Ginger (2 in)
- Water (2 c)
- Carrots (2 chopped)
- Garlic (4 cloves, chopped)
- Red bell pepper (1 chopped)
- Onion (4 chopped)

Ingredients-Masala

- Nutmeg (.25 tsp)
- Paprika (1 T)
- Cardamom (.5 tsp)
- Cloves (3)
- Cinnamon (.5 tsp)
- Cumin (1 T)
- Coriander (1 T)
- Fenugreek seeds (1 T)
- Turmeric (1 T)
-

Ingredients-Masala

- Red bell peppers (2 chunks)
- Curry gravy (3 c)
- Paneer (16 oz)
- Almond milk (.5 c)
- Red chili powder (1 tsp)
- Plain Greek Yoghurt (.3 c)
- Sea salt (1 tsp)
- Coriander (.3 c chopped)
- Milk (.25 cups)
- Arrowroot powder (.5 tsp)

Cooking instructions

- Add the ingredients for the masala mixture, along with the olive oil to a Dutch oven that is a minimum of 6 quarts and then provide the oven with a medium/low heat.

- Cook the spices for 2 minutes which should be enough for them to start to become fragrant. Add in the garlic along with the ginger and let everything cook for approximately 30 seconds and then add in the onions, red bell pepper and carrots and cook everything for an additional 3 minutes.

- Once all the vegetables have cooked, add in the chopped tomatoes along with the water and let the mixture come to a boil. Once this occurs, turn the heat to low and let it simmer for 30 minutes.

- Add the results to an emersion blender and blend until it takes on the consistency of sauce.

- Separately, combine the red chili powder, sea salt, milk, arrowroot powder and plain Greek yoghurt together in a mixing bowl and, after combining thoroughly, add in 3 cups of curry gravy and mix well.

- Place the results into a pan before adding in the paneer along with the red pepper. All the contents of the pan to boil before turning the heat to medium/low and letting everything cook for 15 minutes.

- Turn off the heat before adding in the coriander prior to serving.

Dessert: Fruit and Seed Medley

For this recipe, you will need to set aside 5 minutes for preparation, 0 minutes of cooking time and the results will feed 1.

Nutrition Information
228 calories
5 g of protein
10 mg of sodium
1 g of fiber
3 g of fat (saturated)
25 g of carbs
13 g of fat

Ingredients

- Pomegranate seeds (.5 oz)
- Flax seeds (.5 oz)
- Dried blueberries (2 T)
- Chia seeds (.5 oz)

Cooking instructions

- Add the chia seeds, dried blueberries, pomegranate seeds and flax seeds together in a small bag and shake well.
- Shake again prior to eating and enjoy.

Chapter 7: Day 4

Breakfast: Protein Bomb

For this recipe, you will need to set aside 12 minutes for preparation, 0 minutes of cooking time and the results will feed 1.

Nutrition Information

206 calories

9 g of protein

237 mg of sodium

1 g of fiber

0 g of fat (saturated)

338 g of carbs

2 g of fat

Ingredients

- Reduced fat cheddar cheese (1 oz)
- Whole grain crackers (5)
- Egg (1)

Cooking instructions

- Place the egg into a small pot before adding in enough cold water to ensure that it is completely submerged in 1 in of cold water.

- Place the pot onto the stove over a burner set to a medium/high heat and allow the water in the pot to come to a boil.
- Once the water has boiled, remove the pot from the stove and allow 10 minutes for it to cool completely before draining the pot.
- Add cold water to a small bowl and dunk the egg in it prior to peeling for an easier time of it.
- Remove the shell from the egg and slice it into 5 bite sized sections. Place each section onto a cracker and top with cheese prior to serving.

Lunch: Stir Fried shrimp

For this recipe, you will need to set aside 30 minutes for preparation, 25 minutes of cooking time and the results will feed 4.

Nutrition Information
292 calories
42.9 g of protein
752 mg of sodium
5 g of fiber
2 g of fat (saturated)
17.5 g of carbs
5.5 g of fat

Ingredients

- Deveined shrimp (1.5 lb peeled)
- Green beans (1 lb)
- Miso (2 T)
- Ginger root (3 in peeled, minced)
- Broccoli (1 head florets)
- Rice wine vinegar (.25 c)
- Chives (1 bunch minced)
- Sesame oil (2 T)

Cooking instructions

- Fill a large pot half full of water and place it on top of the stove over a burner set to a high heat. Allow the water to boil and then add in the green beans along with the broccoli before covering and letting the pot simmer on a low heat for 10 minutes.
- While the pot is simmering, use the sesame oil to coat your skillet and then add in the vinegar, miso, chives and ginger root and placing the skill on top of the stove over a burner set to a medium/low heat.
- Let the ingredients in the skillet cook for 10 minutes prior to adding in the shrimp. Let the shrimp cook for 5 minutes. Once the shrimp begin to curl and turn opaque flip them and cook for another 5 minutes.
- Combine all of the ingredients prior to serving.

Dinner: Cauliflower and Spicy Noodles

For this recipe, you will need to set aside 20 minutes for preparation, 13 minutes of cooking time and the results will feed 4.

Nutrition Information

324 calories

6 g of protein

1037 mg of sodium

4 g of fiber

2 g of fat (saturated)

48 g of carbs

15 g of fat

Ingredients-Sauce

- Rice wine vinegar (2 T)
- Soy sauce (4 T)
- Unrefined sugar (2 T)
- Ketchup (2 T)
- Arrowroot powder (3 tsp)
- Water (.25 cups)

Ingredients-Meal

- Raw cashews (.3 c)
- Garlic (2 cloves minced)
- Yellow pepper (1diced)
- Rice noodles (1 lb)

- Red pepper flakes (1 tsp)
- Olive oil (2 T)
- Orange pepper (1 diced)
- Scallion (5)
- Cauliflower (1 head, florets)

<u>Cooking instructions</u>
- Prepare the noodles as per the instructions on the packaging.
- Using a small bowl, combine the unrefined sugar, .25 cups water, ketchup, arrowroot powder, rice wine vinegar and soy sauce together and mix well.
- Spread the olive oil onto your skillet before place it on the stove on top of a burner set to a medium heat. Add in the cauliflower and let it cook 5 minutes, stirring regularly. Remove the cauliflower from the skillet.
- Place the yellow pepper, red pepper and orange pepper into the skillet and allow them to cook for about 3 minutes before placing the cauliflower back into the skillet and letting everything cook for 5 minutes.
- Add in the ginger, garlic and cashews before letting everything cook for 2 minutes and then adding in the sauce.
- Increase the heat beneath the skillet to high and allow the sauce to thicken for 60 seconds.
- Combine the spring onions with the noodles and top with the sauce prior to serving.

Dessert: Cranberry Scones

For this recipe, you will need to set aside 20 minutes for preparation, 20 minutes of cooking time and the results will feed 8.

Nutrition Information

308 calories

6 g of protein

350 mg of sodium

5 g of fiber

1.5 g of fat (saturated)

38 g of carbs

15 g of fat

Ingredients

- Pecans (1 c chopped)
- Salt (.5 tsp)
- Orange zest (1 tsp grated)
- Canola oil (2 T)
- Unsweetened cranberries (.5 c)
- Baking powder (2 tsp)
- Low fat vanilla yogurt (1.25 cups)
- Baking soda (.5 tsp)
- Whole wheat pastry flour (2 c)

Cooking instructions

- Prepare your oven by heating it to 400 degrees F
- Take a 9 in baking pan and coat it with a cooking spray
- Combine the baking soda, salt, baking powder, whole wheat pastry flour and the pecans in a mixing bowl and mix thoroughly.
- Separately, place the vanilla yogurt, orange zest and oil together and whisk briskly.
- Form a place for the wet ingredients in the bowl of dry ingredients and combine the two bowls before adding in the cranberries and blending just enough for all the ingredients to begin to come together.
- Add the contents of the bowl to the 9 in baking pan and then form 8 triangles from the dough using a sharp knife.
- Place the pan in the oven and let the dough bake for 20 minutes. The scones are ready once you can stick a toothpick through the middle of the middle scone and withdraw it cleanly.
- Allow the scones to cool for 5 minutes before eating.

Chapter 8: Day 5

Breakfast: Scallions and Corn Muffins

For this recipe, you will need to set aside 30 minutes for preparation, 25 minutes of cooking time and the results will feed 4.

Nutrition Information

345 calories

9 g of protein

491 mg of sodium

4 g of fiber

1.5 g of fat (saturated)

47 g of carbs

16 g of fat

Ingredients

- Egg (1)
- Brown sugar (2 tsp)
- Egg whites (2)
- Corn kernels (.75 c)
- Salt (.5 tsp)
- Black pepper (to taste)
- Sea salt (1 pinch)
- Fat free plain Greek Yoghurt (1 c)
- Whole wheat pastry flour (.5 c)
- Red bell pepper (1 chopped)

- Yellow cornmeal (1.5 cups)
- Canola oil (2.5 c +2 T divided)
- Scallions (4 thinly sliced)

Cooking instructions

- Prepare your oven by heating it to 350 degrees F and prepare a muffin tin with muffin cups.
- Add the 2 T of canola oil to a skillet before setting it on top of the stove above a burner set to a medium heat.
- Add the bell pepper to the skillet and allow it to cook for 5 minutes. Add the scallions to the skillet and allow them to cook for 1 minute stirring as needed. Remove the skillet from the stove and allow the contents to cool for 5 minutes.
- While the scallions and bell pepper cook, mix together the flour, baking soda, baking powder, black pepper and cornmeal in a mixing bowl.
- Separately, add the remainder of the canola oil along with the egg, egg whites, yoghurt and sugar to another mixing bowl and whisk well. Add in the corn and the bell pepper before combining the two bowls and folding in the dry ingredients until they begin to get moist.
- Add the resulting concoction to the muffin tin and then place the tin in the oven to allow it to bake for 25 minutes. You will know when the muffins are done when you can stick a toothpick into the middle of the middle muffin and pull it out cleanly.

- Allow the muffins to cool for 5 minutes prior to serving.

Lunch: Kidney Bean Salad with Cucumber, Red Peppers and Corn

For this recipe, you will need to set aside 15 minutes for preparation, 0 minutes of cooking time and the results will feed 4.

Nutrition Information
274 calories
10 g of protein
24 mg of sodium
12 g of fiber
2.3 g of fat (saturated)
38 g of carbs
15 g of fat

Ingredients

- Lime (1)
- Corn (1.25 c)
- Red pepper (1 diced)
- Kidney beans (1 can)
- Salt (as needed)
- Black pepper (as needed)
- English cucumber (1 diced)
- Cilantro (.5 c)
- Avocado (1 peeled, diced)

- Cherry tomatoes (1 c)

<u>Cooking instructions</u>

- Using a salad bowl, combine the kidney beans, cherry tomatoes, cilantro, cucumber, red pepper and corn before adding the lime juice and mixing well.
- Mix in the avocado and season as desired with pepper and salt prior to serving.

Dinner: Spicy Quinoa Casserole

For this recipe, you will need to set aside 20 minutes for preparation, 90 minutes of cooking time and the results will feed 8.

Nutrition Information
601 calories
37.5 g of protein
797 mg of sodium
14 g of fiber
6.5 g of fat (saturated)
82 g of carbs
15 g of fat

<u>Ingredients</u>

- Taco seasoning (1 T)
- Sea salt (1.5 tsp)
- Cilantro (.25 c)

- Mozzarella cheese (16 oz)
- Tomatoes (1 lb chopped)
- Hot water (4 c)
- Green onions (6 chopped)
- Corn kernels (8 oz)
- Black beans (15 oz)
- Quinoa (3 c)

Cooking instructions

- Prepare your oven by heating it to 3350 degrees F.
- Using a 9x13 rectangular baking dish add in the sea sat, cilantro, taco season, tomatoes, green onions, quinoa, hot water, corn kernels and mozzarella cheese.
- Use aluminum foil to cover the dish and place it into the oven to cook for 60 minutes.
- Remove the dish from the oven, uncover it, add the rest of the cheese and place it back in the oven to bake for 30 additional minutes.
- Prepare your broiler and place the pan near it to broil for 2 minutes to allow the top of the casserole to brown.
- Serve hot and enjoy

Dessert: Ginger and Pecan Oatmeal

For this recipe, you will need to set aside 10 minutes for preparation, 5 minutes of cooking time and the results will feed 1.

Nutrition Information

200 calories

6 g of protein

15 mg of sodium

3 g of fiber

2 g of fat (saturated)

30 g of carbs

12 g of fat

Ingredients

- Apple juice (.5 c)
- Steel cut oats (.25 c)
- Grapefruit (.5)
- Pecans (1 T chopped)
- Ginger snap (1 crumbled)

Cooking instructions

- Combine the apple juice along with the water in a small saucepan and set it onto the stove over a burner turned to a high heat and allow it to boil.
- Add the oats to the saucepan before reducing the heat to low and allowing the contents of the pan to simmer for 5 minutes, stirring constantly.
- Allow the oatmeal to sit for 2 minutes prior to topping with the gingersnap and pecans and serving.

Chapter 9: Day 6

Breakfast: Oatmeal with Walnuts

For this recipe, you will need to set aside 10 minutes for preparation, 5 minutes of cooking time and the results will feed 4.

Nutrition Information
353 calories
11 g of protein
70 mg of sodium
6 g of fiber
1.5 g of fat (saturated)
57 g of carbs
12 g of fat

Ingredients

- Rolled oats (1.25 c)
- Walnuts (.5 c chopped)
- Unsweetened dried cranberries (.25 c)
- Milk (2.5 c divided)
- Salt (1 tsp)
- Dried goji berries (.25 c)
- Brown sugar (2 tsp)
- Water (1 c)
- Granny smith apple (1 cored)
- Pear (1 quartered)

<u>Cooking instructions</u>

- Combine 1.5 cups of the milk and the water in a saucepan before adding the saucepan to the stove above a burner that has been turned to a high heat.

- Let the water boil before adding in the oats along with the salt and reducing the heat to medium/low to allow the oats to simmer for 3 minutes. Stir regularly to encourage the oats to soften.

- Add in the pear along with the apple before covering the pan and letting everything simmer for three minutes until the fruit tenderizes. Add in the cranberries along with the goji berries before taking the pan off of the burner and letting it sit, covered, for 60 seconds.

- Split the oatmeal into 4 bowls and cover each with 2 T walnuts, .25 cups milk and .5 tsp sugar.

- Serve hot and enjoy.

Lunch: Avocado and Chicken Salad

For this recipe, you will need to set aside 5 minutes for preparation, 0 minutes of cooking time and the results will feed 1.

Nutrition Information
425 calories
39.6 g of protein
405 mg of sodium
8.5 g of fiber

1 g of fat (saturated)

34 g of carbs

15 g of fat

Ingredients

- Shredded chicken (.75 cups cooked)
- Plain Greek yoghurt (2 T)
- English muffin (1)
- Avocado (.25 peeled, sliced)
- Lemon juice (1 tsp)
- Sunflower sprouts (1 handful)
- Tomato (.25 sliced)

Cooking instructions

- Place the avocado is a small bowl and mash it to form a paste before mixing in the plain Greek yoghurt and the lemon juice.
- Add in the chicken and mix well in order to coat it completely
- Plate the English muffin before topping with the sprouts and the chicken prior to serving.

Dinner: Bean Burger

For this recipe, you will need to set aside 30 minutes for preparation, 30 minutes of cooking time and the results will feed 8.

Nutrition Information

165 calories

4 g of protein

462 mg of sodium

3 g of fiber

1.5 g of fat (saturated)

16.5 g of carbs

10.4 g of fat

Ingredients

- Corn kernels (.5 c)
- Salt (.5 tsp)
- Tomato paste (1 T)
- Paprika (2 tsp)
- Mayonnaise (.25 c)
- Olive oil (4 T)
- Egg (1)
- Basil (1 oz)
- Mayonnaise (.25 c)
- Broth (1 c)
- Baked beans (14 oz)
- Organic farro (.3 c)

Cooking instructions

- Soak the farro overnight to ensure it is easy to cook, drain the water from it prior to cooking.

- Place the broth and the faro into a pot and then place the pot on top of a burner set to a high heat. Once the broth boils, turn the heat to medium/low and let the farro cook for 30 minutes.
- Let the farrow cool before adding all of the ingredients to a mixing bowl and mixing well.
- Form patties from .3 cups of the mixture.
- Add the oil to a skillet before placing the skillet onto a burner turned to a medium heat. Cook the patties for 3 minutes per side.

Dessert: Peanut Butter Bars

For this recipe, you will need to set aside 30 minutes for preparation, 45 seconds of cooking time and the results will feed 6.

Nutrition Information
168 calories
12 g of protein
327 mg of sodium
2 g of fiber
3 g of fat (saturated)
30 g of carbs
16 g of fat

Ingredients

- Cooked rice (1 c)
- Peanut butter (.25 c)
- Maple syrup (2 T)

Cooking instructions

- Add the peanut butter to a bowl that can be microwaved before microwaving it for 45 seconds.
- Combine the maple syrup, rice and peanut butter in a small mixing bowl and mix well.
- Place the peanut butter mixture into an 8x8 glass container and then place the container in the refrigerator to harden for 30 minutes.
- Cut the bars and consume quickly when removed from the refrigerator to prevent the bars from melting.

Chapter 10: Day 7

Breakfast: Smoked Salmon Frittata with Scallions

For this recipe, you will need to set aside 10 minutes for preparation, 15 minutes of cooking time and the results will feed 6.

Nutrition Information
366 calories
10 g of protein
5335 mg of sodium
0 g of fiber
2.5 g of fat (saturated)
1 g of carbs
15 g of fat

Ingredients

- Tarragon (.5 tsp dried)
- Smoked salmon (2 oz)
- Eggs (4)
- Black olive tapenade (.5 c)
- Scallions (6 chopped)
- Water (.25 c)
- Salt (.5 tsp)
- Egg whites (6)
- Extra virgin olive oil (2 tsp)

<u>Cooking instructions</u>

- Prepare your oven by heating it to 350 degrees F.
- Place the olive oil in a skillet and place the skillet on top of a burner turned to a medium heat. Let the oil heat for 25 seconds and then add in the scallions before letting them cook for 2 minutes, stirring regularly.
- In a small bowl, mix together the eggs, egg whites, water, tarragon and salt and whisk well before seasoning with black pepper.
- Add the contents of the bowl to the skillet and then add in the salmon. Cook all of the ingredients for an addition 2 minutes making sure to stir regularly.
- Add the skillet to the oven and bake for 12 minutes
- Place the tapenade on top before serving.

Lunch: Veggie Burger

For this recipe, you will need to set aside 30 minutes for preparation, 15 minutes of cooking time and the results will feed 6.

Nutrition Information
202 calories
7 g of protein
222 mg of sodium
6 g of fiber
1 g of fat (saturated)
30 g of carbs

6 g of fat

Ingredients

- Parsley (2 T)
- Quinoa (.25 c)
- Barley (.25 c)
- Sweet potato (1)
- Cayenne pepper (1 tsp)
- Garbanzo beans (15 oz)
- Black pepper (.5 tsp)
- Cumin (1.5 tsp)
- Salt (.5 tsp)
- Red peppers (1.5)
- Whole wheat flour (2 T)
- Olive oil (2 T)

Cooking instructions

- Prepare your oven by heating it to 400 degrees F
- Place the sweet potato on a baking tray and place the tray in the oven to bake for 45 minutes until it is nice and soft.
- While the sweet potato is baking, place the quinoa and the barely into two different pots filled with boiling water and let both cook for approximately 40 minutes.
- While the potato is roasting, prepare the red peppers and quarter them before placing them in the oven to roast for 15 minutes.

- Remove the sweet potato from the oven and let it cool before adding it, along with the parsley, cayenne pepper, flour, black pepper, cumin, salt and 1 T oil into a food processor and process well.
- Place the results in a mixing bowl before adding in the barley and quinoa after they have cooled.
- Place the remaining oil into a skillet before placing the skillet onto the stove above a burner set to a medium heat.
- Place spoonfuls of the bean mix into the skillet and flatten them into patties. Each side of the patty will require approximately 2 minutes to brown properly.
- Place each patty onto a whole-wheat bun and top with roasted peppers before serving.

Dinner: Samosa Stir Fry

For this recipe, you will need to set aside 10 minutes for preparation, 15 minutes of cooking time and the results will feed 4.

Nutrition Information
308 calories
8.4 g of protein
536 mg of sodium
9 g of fiber
1.1 g of fat (saturated)
39 g of carbs
7.5 g of fat

Ingredients

- Sea salt (1 tsp)
- Onion (1 chopped)
- Ginger (2 T chopped)
- Cilantro (.25 cups chopped)
- Baby potatoes (2 lb)
- Peas (1 cup)
- Coriander (2 tsp)
- Olive oil (2 T)
- Garam masala (2 tsp)

Cooking instructions

- Fill a pot 50 percent of the way full of water before placing it on top of a burner turned to a high heat. After the water boils, add in the potatoes and add extra water if they are not submerged by about an inch of water all the way around. Let them cook on the burner for 10 minutes.
- While the potatoes cook, add the olive oil to a skillet before adding in the ginger along with the onion. After the potatoes finish cooking add them in as well.
- Place the skillet on top of a burner turned to a high/medium heat and all the contents of the skillet to cook for 3 minutes, stirring twice a minute. Mix in the spice, peas and salt before cooking an additional 60 seconds.
- Remove the skillet from the stove, mix in the cilantro and serve.

Dessert: Savory Nut clusters

For this recipe, you will need to set aside 10 minutes for preparation, 10 minutes of cooking time and the results will feed 4.

Nutrition Information

200 calories

6 g of protein

287 mg of sodium

4.5 g of fiber

2 g of fat (saturated)

32 g of carbs

12 g of fat

Ingredients

- Salt (.5 tsp)
- Honey (2.5 T)
- Coconut oil (1 T)
- Raw almonds (2 c)
- Maple syrup (1 T)
- Cayenne pepper (.25 tsp)
- Red pepper flakes (1 tsp)

Cooking instructions

- Prepare your oven by heating it to 350 degrees F
- Using a mixing bowl, combine the honey, maple syrup, almonds, coconut oil, cayenne pepper, salt and red

pepper flakes and mix thoroughly to ensure the almonds are well coated.

- Add the almonds to a baking sheet that you have lined with parchment paper before placing the sheet into the oven for 10 minutes. Stir the almonds after 5 minutes to ensure they are well baked.
- Let the almonds cool for 20 minutes to give the glaze time to set prior to serving.

Chapter 11: Green Smoothie Recipes

Ultimate Detox Smoothies

Kombucha and Spinach Smoothie

This recipe can be ready in 5 minutes, makes 1 serving (24 oz.), and will take approximately 45 seconds of blending assuming you are using a blender that is 1000 watts.

Nutrition Information

334 calories

22 g of fat

10 g of fat (saturated)

35 g of carbs

187 mg of sodium

10 g of fiber

18 g of sugar

3 g of protein

Ingredients

- Kale (1 c)
- Coconut oil (.5 T)
- Kombucha (1 c)
- Frozen papaya (.5 c)
- Cinnamon (.5 tsp)
- Spinach (1 c)
- Honey (.5 T)

- Flax seed (1 T)
- Ginger (2 tsp)

Cayenne and Arugula Smoothie

This recipe can be ready in 5 minutes, makes 1 serving (24 oz.), and will take approximately 45 seconds of blending assuming you are using a blender that is 1000 watts.

Nutrition Information
260 calories
2 g of fat
0 g of fat (saturated)
50 g of carbs
50 mg of sodium
13 g of fiber
30 g of sugar
4 g of protein

Ingredients
- Maca (.5 T)
- Flax seed (1 T ground)
- Cayenne pepper (.25 tsp)
- Pear (1 halved)
- Honey (.5 tsp)
- Green apple (1 cored)
- Arugula (.5 c)
- Ginger (.5 tsp)

- Kale (1 c)
- Dandelion greens (1 c)
- Water (1 c)
- Lemon juice (.5 c)

Spicy Hot Smoothie

This recipe can be ready in 5 minutes, makes 1 serving (24 oz.), and will take approximately 45 seconds of blending assuming you are using a blender that is 1000 watts.

Nutrition Information
340 calories
24 g of fat
0 g of fat (saturated)
32 g of carbs
175 mg of sodium
12 g of fiber
15 g of sugar
5 g of protein

Ingredients
- Water (1 c)
- Kale (1 c)
- Frozen blueberries (.5 c)
- Avocado (.5 peeled)
- Coconut oil (.5 T)
- Chia seeds (1 T)

- Honey (.5 T)
- Chili powder (.25 tsp)
- Protein powder (20 g)
- Coconut flakes (1 T)
- Plain Greek yoghurt (.25 c)
- Maca (1 T)

Flax Seed and Kale Smoothie

This recipe can be ready in 5 minutes, makes 1 serving (24 oz.), and will take approximately 45 seconds of blending assuming you are using a blender that is 1000 watts.

Nutrition Information
275 calories
13 g of fat
5 g of fat (saturated)
40 g of carbs
285 mg of sodium
13 g of fiber
17 g of sugar
6 g of protein

Ingredients
- Frozen banana (1 peeled)
- Coconut oil (.5 T)
- Almond milk (1 c)
- Kale (1 c)

- Cinnamon (.25 tsp)
- Coconut flakes (1 T)
- Honey (.5 T)
- Flax seed (1 T)
- Protein powder (20 g)

Cacao and Avocado Smoothie

This recipe can be ready in 5 minutes, makes 1 serving (24 oz.), and will take approximately 45 seconds of blending assuming you are using a blender that is 1000 watts.

Nutrition Information
260 calories
15 g of fat
3 g of fat (saturated)
30 g of carbs
400 mg of sodium
9 g of fiber
17 g of sugar
7 g of protein

Ingredients
- Spirulina powder (1 T)
- Water (1 c)
- Spinach (1 c)
- Avocado (.5 peeled)
- Cinnamon (.25 tsp)

- Cacao powder (.5 T)
- Honey (.5 T)
- Pink Himalayan salt (1 tsp)
- Flax seed (1 T)
- Maca (.5 T)
- Protein powder (20 g)

Watermelon and Turmeric Smoothie

This recipe can be ready in 5 minutes, makes 1 serving (24 oz.), and will take approximately 45 seconds of blending assuming you are using a blender that is 1000 watts.

Nutrition Information
182 calories
1 gram of fat
0 g of fat (saturated)
45 g of carbs
285 mg of sodium
13 g of fiber
25 g of sugar
4 g of protein

Ingredients
- Frozen banana (1 peeled)
- Dandelion greens (1 c chopped)
- Water (.5 c)
- Watermelon (1 cup fresh)

- Cinnamon (.25 tsp)
- Honey (.5 T)
- Line juice (.5 lime)
- Ginger (.5 T)
- Turmeric (.5 tsp)
- Lemon juice (.5 lemons)

Dandelion and Banana Smoothie

This recipe can be ready in 5 minutes, makes 1 serving (24 oz.), and will take approximately 45 seconds of blending assuming you are using a blender that is 1000 watts.

Nutrition Information
230 calories
1 gram of fat
0 g of fat (saturated)
59 g of carbs
55 mg of sodium
10 g of fiber
34 g of sugar
3 g of protein

Ingredients
- Chia seeds (1 T)
- Coconut oil (1 tsp)
- Spinach (.5 c)
- Coconut flakes (1 T)

- Water (1 c)
- Lemon (.5)
- Frozen banana (1 peeled)
- Red apple (1 cored)
- Dandelion greens (.5 c)

Green Tea and Spinach Smoothie

This recipe can be ready in 5 minutes, makes 1 serving (24 oz.), and will take approximately 45 seconds of blending assuming you are using a blender that is 1000 watts.

Nutrition Information
175 calories
5 g of fat
0 g of fat (saturated)
34 g of carbs
76 mg of sodium
4 g of fiber
20 g of sugar
15 g of protein

Ingredients
- Frozen banana (1 peeled)
- Baby spinach (1 c)
- Brewed green tea (1 cup)
- Honey (1 tsp)
- Protein powder (20 g)

- Honey (1 tsp)

Strawberry Arugula Smoothie

This recipe can be ready in 5 minutes, makes 1 serving (24 oz.), and will take approximately 45 seconds of blending assuming you are using a blender that is 1000 watts.

Nutrition Information
174 calories
5 g of fat
0 g of fat (saturated)
33 g of carbs
133 mg of sodium
5 g of fiber
18 g of sugar
2 g of protein

<u>Ingredients</u>
- Frozen banana (1 peeled)
- Arugula (.5 c)
- Frozen strawberries (1 c)
- Water (1 c)
- Spinach (.5 c)
- Sea salt (1 tsp)
- Honey (.5 T)
- Coconut oil (1 tsp)

Kale and Lime Smoothie

This recipe can be ready in 5 minutes, makes 1 serving (24 oz.), and will take approximately 45 seconds of blending assuming you are using a blender that is 1000 watts.

Nutrition Information

191 calories

1 g of fat

0 g of fat (saturated)

50 g of carbs

35 mg of sodium

5 g of fiber

30 g of sugar

3 g of protein

Ingredients

- Lemon (.5 peeled)
- Frozen banana (1 peeled)
- Ginger (.25 inch)
- Water (1 c)
- Pink Himalayan salt (1 tsp)
- Lime (.5 peeled)
- Kale (1 c)
- Honey (1 T)

Mango and Avocado Smoothie

This recipe can be ready in 5 minutes, makes 1 serving (24 oz.), and will take approximately 45 seconds of blending assuming you are using a blender that is 1000 watts.

Nutrition Information

240 calories

15 g of fat

3 g of fat (saturated)

30 g of carbs

285 mg of sodium

10 g of fiber

16 g of sugar

3 g of protein

Ingredients

- Frozen mango (.5 c)
- Spinach (.5 c)
- Honey (.5 T)
- Cinnamon (.5 tsp)
- Flax seed (1 T)
- Avocado (.5 peeled)
- Frozen blueberries (.5 cups)
- Arugula (.5 c)
- Kale (.5 cups)

Dandelion Greens and Mixed Berry Smoothie

This recipe can be ready in 5 minutes, makes 1 serving (24 oz.), and will take approximately 45 seconds of blending assuming you are using a blender that is 1000 watts.

Nutrition Information
270 calories
15 g of fat
9 g of fat (saturated)
36 g of carbs
75 mg of sodium
7 g of fiber
19 g of sugar
18 g of protein

Ingredients

- Honey (.5 T)
- Frozen blackberries (1 c)
- Coconut oil (1 T)
- Flax seed (1 T)
- Frozen banana (1 peeled)
- Cinnamon (.25 tsp)
- Coconut oil (1 T)
- Water (1 c)
- Dandelion greens (1 c)

Baby Spinach and Pear Smoothie

This recipe can be ready in 5 minutes, makes 1 serving (24 oz.), and will take approximately 45 seconds of blending assuming you are using a blender that is 1000 watts.

Nutrition Information

222 calories

8 g of fat

0 g of fat (saturated)

39 g of carbs

24 mg of sodium

8 g of fiber

26 g of sugar

3 g of protein

Ingredients

- Pear (1 peeled)
- Flax seed (1 T)
- Baby spinach (1 c)
- Water (1 c)
- Ginger (.5 tsp)
- Honey (.5 T)
- Water (1 c)
- Flax seed (1 T)

Spicy Spinach Smoothie

This recipe can be ready in 5 minutes, makes 1 serving (24 oz.), and will take approximately 45 seconds of blending assuming you are using a blender that is 1000 watts.

Nutrition Information

170 calories

8 g of fat

1 g of fat (saturated)

28 g of carbs

300 mg of sodium

4 g of fiber

15 g of sugar

2 g of protein

Ingredients

- Frozen banana (1 peeled)
- Coconut oil (.5 T)
- Honey (.5 T)
- Chili powder (.25 tsp)
- Water (1 c)
- Spinach (1 c)
- Cayenne pepper (.25 tsp)
- Flax seed (1 T)

Romaine Lettuce and Ginger Smoothie

This recipe can be ready in 5 minutes, makes 1 serving (32 oz.), and will take approximately 45 seconds of blending assuming you are using a blender that is 1000 watts.

Nutrition Information

135 calories

4 g of fat

0 g of fat (saturated)

60 g of carbs

85 mg of sodium

1 g of fiber

24 g of sugar

9 g of protein

Ingredients

- Romaine lettuce (3 c)
- Ginger (.25 inches)
- Frozen mango (1 pitted)
- Lemons (2 peeled)
- Chia seeds (2 T)
- Spinach (2 c)
- Water (1 c)

Radish and Greens Smoothie

This recipe can be ready in 5 minutes, makes 1 serving (32 oz.), and will take approximately 45 seconds of blending assuming you are using a blender that is 1000 watts.

Nutrition Information
373 calories
2 g of fat
0 g of fat (saturated)
60 g of carbs
35 mg of sodium
15 g of fiber
16 g of sugar
6 g of protein

Ingredients
- Tangerines (2 peeled)
- Radish greens (1.5 c)
- Water (1 c)
- Red apple (1 cored)
- Dandelion greens (1 c)
- Ginger (.5 tsp)

Chard and Banana Smoothie

This recipe can be ready in 5 minutes, makes 1 serving (24 oz.), and will take approximately 45 seconds of blending assuming you are using a blender that is 1000 watts.

Nutrition Information

200 calories

13 g of fat

2 g of fat (saturated)

35 g of carbs

109 mg of sodium

8 g of fiber

22 g of sugar

10 g of protein

Ingredients

- Frozen banana (1 peeled)
- Almond butter (1 T)
- Mixed greens (2 c)
- Almond milk (.5 cups)

Kiwi Celery Smoothie

This recipe can be ready in 5 minutes, makes 1 serving (24 oz.), and will take approximately 45 seconds of blending assuming you are using a blender that is 1000 watts.

Nutrition Information

150 calories

9 g of fat

0 g of fat (saturated)

45 g of carbs

67 mg of sodium

15 g of fiber

22 g of sugar

11 g of protein

<u>Ingredients</u>

- Spinach (2 c)
- Pineapple (.25 cups)
- Kiwi (1 peeled)
- Water (1 c)
- Celery (2 stalks)
- Frozen banana (1)

Spinach and Mixed Berry Smoothie

This recipe can be ready in 5 minutes, makes 1 serving (24 oz.), and will take approximately 45 seconds of blending assuming you are using a blender that is 1000 watts.

Nutrition Information

275 calories

13 g of fat

5 g of fat (saturated)

40 g of carbs

285 mg of sodium

13 g of fiber

17 g of sugar

6 g of protein

Ingredients

- Spinach (2 c)
- Red apple (1 cored)
- Almond milk (1 c)
- Mixed berries (1 c)

Banana, Spinach and Pineapple Smoothie

This recipe can be ready in 5 minutes, makes 1 serving (24 oz.), and will take approximately 45 seconds of blending assuming you are using a blender that is 1000 watts.

Nutrition Information

300 calories

12 g of fat

2 g of fat (saturated)

22 g of carbs

189 mg of sodium

16 g of fiber

28 g of sugar

11 g of protein

- Spinach (2 c)

- Frozen banana (1 peeled)

- Green apple (1 cored)

- Pineapple (1 c)

- Water (1 c)

Chard and Coconut Smoothie

This recipe can be ready in 5 minutes, makes 1 serving (24 oz.), and will take approximately 45 seconds of blending assuming you are using a blender that is 1000 watts.

Nutrition Information
375 calories
12 g of protein
11 g of fat
4 g of fat (saturated)
28 g of carbs
23 g of sugar
9 g of fiber
54 mg of sodium

Ingredients

- Chard (1 c)

- Plain yoghurt (1 c)

- Frozen strawberries (1 c)

- Frozen banana (1 peeled)

Weight loss smoothies

High Protein Pear Smoothie

This recipe can be ready in 5 minutes, makes 1 serving (24 oz.), and will take approximately 45 seconds of blending assuming you are using a blender that is 1000 watts.

Nutrition Information
299 calories
9 g of fiber
27 g of protein
37 g of carbs
595 mg of sodium
6 g of fat
2 g of fat (saturated)
27 g of sugar

Ingredients
- Almond milk (1 c)
- Spinach (1 c)
- Protein powder (20 g)
- Pear (1 cored)
- Matcha tea (.5 tsp)

Orange Smoothie with Spinach

This recipe can be ready in 5 minutes, makes 1 serving (24 oz.), and will take approximately 45 seconds of blending assuming you are using a blender that is 1000 watts.

Nutrition Information
146 calories
36 g of carbs
3 g of fat
25 g of sugar
100 mg of sodium
4 g of protein
6 g of fiber
0 g of fat (saturated)

Ingredients

- Spinach (1 c tightly packed)
- Navel orange (1 peeled)
- Banana (.5 peeled)
- Coconut water (.25 c)
- Ice cubes (6)
- Hemp seed (1 T)

Orange Protein Smoothie with Kale

This recipe can be ready in 5 minutes, makes 1 serving (24 oz.), and will take approximately 45 seconds of blending assuming you are using a blender that is 1000 watts.

Nutrition Information

300 calories

23 g of sugar

7 g of fiber

613 mg of sodium

35 g of carbs

2 g of fat (saturated)

6 g of fat

30 g of protein

Ingredients

- Water (1 c)
- Kale (1 c chopped)
- Protein powder (20 g)
- Spirulina powder (.5 tsp.)
- Navel orange (1 peeled)
- Cinnamon (1 tsp)
- Ginger (1 tsp powdered)

Green Smoothie with Orange and Ginger

This recipe can be ready in 5 minutes, makes 2 servings (48 oz.), and will take approximately 45 seconds of blending assuming you are using a blender that is 1000 watts.

Nutrition Information

300 calories

40 g of carbs

0 g of fat (saturated)

50 mg of sodium

2 g of fat

12 g of fiber

10 g of protein

28 g of sugar

Ingredients

- Spinach (2 c packed tightly)
- Water (1.5 c)
- Romain lettuce (1 c packed tightly)
- Banana (2 peeled)
- Navel orange (2 peeled)
- Cucumber (1 peeled and chopped)
- Ginger (1 inch)

Green Smoothie with Mint and Blueberries

This recipe can be ready in 5 minutes, makes 1 serving (24 oz.), and will take approximately 45 seconds of blending assuming you are using a blender that is 1000 watts.

Nutrition Information

230 calories

50 g of carbs

5 g of protein

11 g of fiber

35 g of sugar

200 mg of sodium

1.5 g of fat

0 g of fat (saturated)

Ingredients

- Blueberries (2 c)
- Spinach (2 c)
- Mint leaves (4 crushed)
- Kiwi (1 peeled)
- Coconut water (1 c)
- Ice (1 c)

Green Smoothie with Kale and Pineapple

This recipe can be ready in 5 minutes, makes 1 serving (24 oz.), and will take approximately 45 seconds of blending assuming you are using a blender that is 1000 watts.

Nutrition Information

350 calories

8 g of fat

19 g of sugar

12 g of fiber

6 g of protein

3 g of fat (saturated)

45 g of carbs

<u>Ingredients</u>

- Kale (1 c)
- Cucumber (1 c)
- Cilantro (1 c)
- Lemon Juice (1 tsp.)
- Avocado (.5 peeled)

Rolled Oats Breakfast Smoothie

This recipe can be ready in 5 minutes, makes 1 serving (24 oz.), and will take approximately 45 seconds of blending assuming you are using a blender that is 1000 watts.

Nutrition Information
260 calories
8 g of fat
16 g of sugar
40 g of carbs
11 g of protein
6 g of fiber
114 mg of sodium
3 g of fat (saturated)

<u>Ingredients</u>

- Milk (.75 c)
- Banana (1)
- Rolled oats (.25 cups uncooked)
- Spinach (2 c tightly packed)

- Flax seed (2 T)

Honeydew Smoothie with Lime

This recipe can be ready in 5 minutes, makes 4 servings (24 oz. each), and will take approximately 45 seconds of blending assuming you are using a blender that is 1000 watts.

Nutrition Information
240 calories
4 g of protein
15 g of carbs
50 mg of sodium
4 g of fat (saturated)
17 g of sugar
4 g of fiber
9 g of fat

Ingredients
- Honeydew (4 c)
- Mint leaves (1 c)
- Coconut milk (.5 c)
- Ice (1 c)
- Lime juice (1 tsp.)

Peaches and Kale Smoothie

This recipe can be ready in 5 minutes, makes 1 serving (24 oz.), and will take approximately 45 seconds of blending assuming you are using a blender that is 1000 watts.

Nutrition Information
400 calories
34 g of sugar
33 g of protein
2 g of fiber
600 mg of sodium
60 g of carbs
2.5 g of fat (saturated)
9 g of fat

<u>Ingredients</u>
- Frozen peaches (1 c)
- Protein powder (20 g)
- Almond milk (1 c)
- Banana (1 peeled)
- Pineapple (1 c frozen)
- Flaxseed (1 T)
- Kale (2 c)

Pineapple Avocado Smoothie

This recipe can be ready in 5 minutes, makes 2 servings (12 oz. each), and will take approximately 45 seconds of blending assuming you are using a blender that is 1000 watts.

Nutrition Information
169 calories
20 g of carbs
6 g of fat
6 g of sugar
18 g of protein
4 g of fiber
0 g of fat (saturated)
345 mg of sodium

<u>Ingredients</u>

- Kale (2 c packed tightly)
- Almond milk (.5 c)
- Pineapple (.5 c chunked)
- Protein powder (20 g)
- Avocado (.5 peeled)
- Ice cubes (1 c)

Agave, Spinach and Kale Smoothie

This recipe can be ready in 5 minutes, makes 2 servings (24 oz. each), and will take approximately 45 seconds of blending assuming you are using a blender that is 1000 watts.

Nutrition Information

300 calories

80 mg of sodium

5 g of protein

40 g of carbs

8 g of fat (saturated)

9 g of fiber

16 g of sugar

15 g of fat

Ingredients

- Coconut milk (.5 c)
- Coconut water (1 c)
- Agave syrup (1 T)
- Pear (1 peeled, cored)
- Lime juice (1 lime)
- Spinach (2 c)
- Kale (2 c)

Spicy Green Smoothie

This recipe can be ready in 5 minutes, makes 1 serving (24 oz.), and will take approximately 45 seconds of blending assuming you are using a blender that is 1000 watts.

Nutrition Information

260 calories

32 g of carbs

14 g of sugar

4 g of fat (saturated)

12 g of fat

125 mg of sodium

8 g of protein

6 g of fiber

Ingredients

- Cayenne pepper (1 tsp)
- Avocado (.5 peeled)
- Coconut water (1 c)
- Kale (1 c)
- Frozen pineapple (.5 c)
- Spinach (1 c)

Honey and Spinach Smoothie

This recipe can be ready in 5 minutes, makes 1 serving (24 oz.), and will take approximately 45 seconds of blending assuming you are using a blender that is 1000 watts.

Nutrition Information

300 calories

4 g of fat

1 g of fiber

45 g of protein

25 g of carbs

19 g of sugar

2 g of fat (saturated)

140 mg of sodium

Ingredients

- Honey (1 T)
- Spinach (1 c)
- Protein powder (20 grams)
- Ice (1 c)
- Ice water (5 oz)

Apple and Greens Smoothie

This recipe can be ready in 5 minutes, makes 1 serving (24 oz.), and will take approximately 45 seconds of blending assuming you are using a blender that is 1000 watts.

Nutrition Information

290 calories

600 mg of sodium

2 g of fat (saturated)

28 g of protein

34 g of carbs

23 g of sugar

7 g of fiber

6 g of fat

Ingredients

- Kale (1 c)

- Spinach (1 c)
- Almond milk (1 c)
- Cucumber (1 chopped)
- Protein powder (20 g)
- Green apple (1 cored)
- Lemon juice (1 tsp)

Avocado and Lime Smoothie

This recipe can be ready in 5 minutes, makes 1 serving (24 oz.), and will take approximately 45 seconds of blending assuming you are using a blender that is 1000 watts.

Nutrition Information
340 calories
10 g of protein
34 g of carbs
19 g of sugar
9 g of fiber
8 g of fat (saturated)
50 mg of sodium
22 g of fat

Ingredients
- Baby spinach (.5 c)
- Lime (1 peeled)
- Lime zest (1 lime)
- Almond milk (1 c)

- Avocado (.5 peeled)
- Vanilla extract (.5 tsp)
- Honey (.5 T)
- Vanilla extract (.5 tsp)
- Sea salt (1 tsp)

Basil and Chlorella Smoothie

This recipe can be ready in 5 minutes, makes 1 serving (24 oz.), and will take approximately 45 seconds of blending assuming you are using a blender that is 1000 watts.

Nutrition Information
320 calories
240 mg of sodium
15 g of fat
10 g of fiber
4 g of fat (saturated
13 g of protein
35 g of carbs
22 g of sugar

Ingredients
- Frozen pineapple (.5 c chunks)
- Coconut water (1 c)
- Avocado (.5 peeled)
- Basil (6 leaves)
- Plain yoghurt (.25 c)

- Chia seeds (1 tsp)

- Maca (1 tsp)

- Chlorella (1 tsp)

- Lemon juice (1 tsp)

- Bee pollen (1 tsp)

- Sea salt (1 tsp)

- Honey (.5 T)

Berries and Beets Smoothie

This recipe can be ready in 5 minutes, makes 1 serving (24 oz.), and will take approximately 45 seconds of blending assuming you are using a blender that is 1000 watts.

Nutrition Information
280 calories
30 mg of sodium
7 g of fat (saturated)
21 g of sugar
4 g of protein
38 g of carbs
15 g of fiber
15 g of fat

Ingredients

- Coconut oil (1 T)

- Ginger (2 tsp)

- Beet greens (.5 c)

- Beets (.5 c cooked)
- Water (1 c)
- Frozen raspberries (.5 c)
- Lemon (1 peeled)
- Frozen blackberries (.5 c)

Dandelion Smoothie with Lime

This recipe can be ready in 5 minutes, makes 1 serving (24 oz.), and will take approximately 45 seconds of blending assuming you are using a blender that is 1000 watts.

Nutrition Information
190 calories
1 g of fat
43 g of carbs
80 mg of sodium
6 g of fiber
7 g of protein
0 g of fat (saturated)
25 g of sugar

Ingredients
- Lemon juice (1 peeled)
- Frozen banana (1 peeled)
- Water (1 c)
- Spirulina (.5 tsp)
- Dandelion greens (1.5 cups destemmed)

- Chlorella (1 tsp)
- Honey (.5 T)
- Ice cubes (7)
- Pink Himalayan salt (1 tsp)

Avocado and Mango Smoothie

This recipe can be ready in 5 minutes, makes 1 serving (24 oz.), and will take approximately 45 seconds of blending assuming you are using a blender that is 1000 watts.

Nutrition Information
314 calories
16 g of fat
5 g of protein
100 mg of sodium
48 g of carbs
30 g of sugar
3 g of fat (saturated)
11 g of fiber

Ingredients
- Avocado (1 peeled)
- Cilantro (.5 c)
- Water (1 c)
- Frozen mango (1 c)
- Line juice (1 lime)
- Spinach (1 c)

- Ginger (.25 inch)
- Raw honey (.5 T)

Guacamole Smoothie

This recipe can be ready in 5 minutes, makes 1 serving (24 oz.), and will take approximately 45 seconds of blending assuming you are using a blender that is 1000 watts.

Nutrition Information
350 calories
7 g of fat (saturated)
30 g of fat
250 mg of sodium
24 g of carbs
4 g of sugar
15 g of fiber
5 g of protein

<u>Ingredients</u>
- Avocado (1 peeled)
- Tomato (1 c)
- Water (1 c)
- Line juice (.25 c)
- Sea salt (1 tsp)
- Cilantro (.5 c)

Spinach and Strawberry Smoothie

This recipe can be ready in 5 minutes, makes 1 serving (24 oz.), and will take approximately 45 seconds of blending assuming you are using a blender that is 1000 watts.

Nutrition Information

500 calories

200 mg of sodium

8 g of fat (saturated)

15 g of fat

32 g of sugar

45 g of carbs

12 g of protein

13 g of fiber

Ingredients

- Banana (1 peeled)
- Spinach (1 c)
- Almond milk (1.5 c)
- Frozen strawberries (.5 c)
- Plain Greek yogurt (2)
- Frozen mango (.5 c)
- Chia seeds (1 T)
- Bee pollen (1 tsp)
- Coconut oil (1 T)

Immune system boosting smoothies

Cinnamon and Spinach Smoothie

This recipe can be ready in 5 minutes, makes 1 serving (24 oz.), and will take approximately 45 seconds of blending assuming you are using a blender that is 1000 watts.

Nutrition Information
304 calories
105 mg of sodium
15 g of fat
3 g of protein
46 g of carbs
7 g of fiber
20 g of sugar
3 g of fat (saturated)

Ingredients
- Frozen banana (1 peeled)
- Spinach (1 c)
- Water (1 c)
- Frozen blackberries (1 c)
- Basil (5 leaves)
- Cinnamon (.25 tsp)
- Coconut oil (1 T)
- Stevia (1 tsp)

Wheatgrass and Goji Berry Smoothie

This recipe can be ready in 5 minutes, makes 1 serving (24 oz.), and will take approximately 45 seconds of blending assuming you are using a blender that is 1000 watts.

Nutrition Information

500 calories

22 g of fat

15 g of protein

200 mg of sodium

50 g of carbs

29 g of sugar

20 g of fiber

1 gram of fat (saturated)

Ingredients

- Wheatgrass (1 tsp powdered)
- Stevia (1 tsp)
- Coconut oil (1 T)
- Coconut flakes (1 T)
- Maca (1 tsp)
- Dried cranberries (2 T)
- Greek yoghurt (.5 c)
- Goji berries (2 T)
- Kale (.5 c)
- Frozen mango (.5 c)
- Spinach (.5 c)

- Coconut water (1 c)
- Avocado (.5 peeled)

Aloe Vera and Blueberry Smoothie

This recipe can be ready in 5 minutes, makes 1 serving (24 oz.), and will take approximately 45 seconds of blending assuming you are using a blender that is 1000 watts.

Nutrition Information
275 calories
3 g of fat (saturated)
30 g of carbs
7 g of fiber
45 mg of sodium
17 g of fat
3 g of protein
24 g of sugar

Ingredients
- Aloe vera (.5 cups)
- Avocado (.5 peeled)
- Water (1 c)
- Frozen blueberries (.5 c)
- Coconut oil (.5 T)
- Spinach (1 c)
- Pink Himalayan salt (1 T)
- Stevia (.5 tsp)

- Coconut oil (.5 T)

Strawberry Smoothie with Mint

This recipe can be ready in 5 minutes, makes 1 serving (24 oz.), and will take approximately 45 seconds of blending assuming you are using a blender that is 1000 watts.

Nutrition Information
160 calories
20 g of sugar
40 g of carbs
0 g of fat (saturated)
12 g of fiber
3 g of protein
300 mg of sodium
1 g of fat

Ingredients
- Frozen banana (1 peeled)
- Frozen strawberries (1 c)
- Water (1 c)
- Mint leaves (2 c)
- Spinach (1 c)
- Stevia (1 tsp)

Banana and Rosemary Smoothie

This recipe can be ready in 5 minutes, makes 1 serving (24 oz.), and will take approximately 45 seconds of blending assuming you are using a blender that is 1000 watts.

Nutrition Information

200 calories

50 g of carbs

232 mg of sodium

1 gram of fat

29 g of sugar

9 g of fiber

3 g of protein

0 g of fat (saturated)

<u>Ingredients</u>

- Frozen banana (1 peeled)
- Blueberries (1 c)
- Water (1 c)
- Rosemary (2 sprigs)
- Sea salt (1 tsp)
- Stevia (1 tsp)

Beet Greens and Cinnamon Smoothie

This recipe can be ready in 5 minutes, makes 1 serving (24 oz.), and will take approximately 45 seconds of blending assuming you are using a blender that is 1000 watts.

Nutrition Information

200 calories

1 gram of fat

10 g of fiber

75 mg of sodium

25 g of sugar

0 g of fat (saturated)

50 g of carbs

3 g of protein

Ingredients

- Green apple (1 cored)
- Frozen blueberries (.5 c)
- Water (1 c)
- Frozen banana (1 peeled)
- Cinnamon (1 tsp)
- Beet greens (1.5 c)
- Stevia (1 tsp)

Spinach and Mint Smoothie

This recipe can be ready in 5 minutes, makes 1 serving (24 oz.), and will take approximately 45 seconds of blending assuming you are using a blender that is 1000 watts.

Nutrition Information

230 calories

3 g of fat (saturated)

7 g of fiber

75 mg of sodium

23 g of sugar

40 g of carbs

4 g of protein

8 g of fat

Ingredients

- Frozen banana (1 peeled)
- Spinach (1 c)
- Almond milk (1 c)
- Frozen blueberries (1 c)
- Coconut oil (1 T)
- Mint leaves (1 cup)
- Stevia (1 tsp)

Kale Smoothie with Blueberries

This recipe can be ready in 5 minutes, makes 1 serving (24 oz.), and will take approximately 45 seconds of blending assuming you are using a blender that is 1000 watts.

Nutrition Information

367 calories

13 g of fat

75 mg of sodium

25 g of sugar

50 g of carbs

10 g of fiber

20 g of protein

6 g of fat (saturated)

Ingredients

- Frozen blueberries (.5 c)
- Almond milk (1 c)
- Frozen banana (1 peeled)
- Cinnamon (.5 tsp)
- Kale (1 c)
- Stevia (1 tsp)
- Coconut oil (1 T)

Banana and Beets Smoothie

This recipe can be ready in 5 minutes, makes 1 serving (24 oz.), and will take approximately 45 seconds of blending assuming you are using a blender that is 1000 watts.

Nutrition Information

150 calories

3 g of fat

10 g of fiber

25 g of sugar

75 mg of sodium

0 g of fat (saturated)

50 g of carbs

3 g of protein

Ingredients

- Beet greens (1 c chopped)
- Frozen banana (1 peeled)
- Chia seeds (1 T)
- Water (1 c)
- Coconut oil (1 T)
- Stevia (1 tsp)

Mixed Berry and Lettuce Smoothie

This recipe can be ready in 5 minutes, makes 1 serving (24 oz.), and will take approximately 45 seconds of blending assuming you are using a blender that is 1000 watts.

Nutrition Information
190 calories
0 g of fat (saturated)
45 g of carbs
8 g of fiber
25 g of sugar
210 mg of sodium
4 g of protein
1 gram of fat

Ingredients

- Red apple (1 cored)
- Cinnamon (.25 tsp)
- Kale (1 cup)

- Water (1 cup)
- Pink Himalayan salt (1 tsp)
- Frozen banana (1 peeled)
- Stevia (1 tsp)

Greens on Greens Smoothie

This recipe can be ready in 5 minutes, makes 1 serving (24 oz.), and will take approximately 45 seconds of blending assuming you are using a blender that is 1000 watts.

Nutrition Information
140 calories
15 g of sugar
2 g of fat
4 g of protein
35 g of carbs
150 mg of sodium
4 g of fiber
0 g of fat (saturated)

Ingredients
- Kale (1 c)
- Baby spinach (1 c)
- Coconut flakes (.25 cups)
- Frozen banana (1 peeled)
- Water (1 c)
- Coconut oil (1 T)

Apples, Apples, Apples Green Smoothie

This recipe can be ready in 5 minutes, makes 1 serving (24 oz.), and will take approximately 45 seconds of blending assuming you are using a blender that is 1000 watts.

Nutrition Information

300 calories

32 g of sugar

9 g of fiber

1 gram of fat (saturated)

300 mg of sodium

60 g of carbs

3 g of protein

5 g of fat

Ingredients

- Red apple (1 cored)
- Green apple (1 cored)
- Yellow apple (1 cored)
- Coconut oil (1 T)
- Baby spinach (1 c)
- Cinnamon (.5 tsp)
- Water (1 c)
- Maca (.5 T)

Banana and Mint Smoothie

This recipe can be ready in 5 minutes, makes 1 serving (24 oz.), and will take approximately 45 seconds of blending assuming you are using a blender that is 1000 watts.

Nutrition Information

280 calories

25 g of sugar

6 g of fiber

0 g of fat (saturated)

75 mg of sodium

35 g of carbs

10 g of protein

12 g of fat

Ingredients

- Frozen blueberries (1 c)
- Chia seeds (1 T)
- Almond milk (1 c)
- Mint leaves (10)
- Frozen banana (1 peeled)
- Water (1 c)
- Stevia (1 tsp)
- Coconut oil (1 T)

Strawberry and Salad Smoothie

This recipe can be ready in 5 minutes, makes 1 serving (24 oz.), and will take approximately 45 seconds of blending assuming you are using a blender that is 1000 watts.

Nutrition Information
200 calories
125 mg of sodium
6 g of fat
7 g of fiber
20 g of sugar
40 g of carbs
0 g of fat (saturated)
3 g of protein

Ingredients

- Frozen strawberries (1 c)
- Sea salt (1 tsp)
- Flax seed (1 T)
- Salad greens (1 c)
- Water (1 c)
- Kale (.5 c)
- Cinnamon (1 tsp)
- Frozen banana (1 peeled)
- Stevia (1 tsp)
- Coconut oil (1 T)

Banana and Romaine Lettuce Smoothie

This recipe can be ready in 5 minutes, makes 1 serving (24 oz.), and will take approximately 45 seconds of blending assuming you are using a blender that is 1000 watts.

Nutrition Information

160 calories

0 g of fat (saturated)

6 g of fiber

3 g of protein

40 g of carbs

1 g of fat

20 g of sugar

289 mg of sodium

Ingredients

- Frozen pineapple (.5 c)
- Frozen mango (.5 c)
- Romaine lettuce (2 c chopped)
- Chia seeds (1 T)
- Water (1 c)
- Coconut flakes (1 T)
- Coconut oil (1 T)
- Stevia (1 tsp)
- Frozen banana (1 peeled)

Kiwi and Spinach Smoothie

This recipe can be ready in 5 minutes, makes 1 serving (24 oz.), and will take approximately 45 seconds of blending assuming you are using a blender that is 1000 watts.

Nutrition Information
150 calories
25 g of sugar
0 g of fat (saturated)
3 g of protein
50 g of carbs
75 mg of sodium
3 g of fat
10 g of fiber

<u>Ingredients</u>

- Frozen banana (1 peeled)
- Spinach (1 c)
- Pink Himalayan salt (1 tsp)
- Kiwi (2 peeled)
- Chia seeds (1 T)
- Water (1 c)
- Coconut flakes (1 T)
- Coconut oil (1 T)
- Stevia (1 tsp)

Kale and Green Apple Smoothie

This recipe can be ready in 5 minutes, makes 1 serving (24 oz.), and will take approximately 45 seconds of blending assuming you are using a blender that is 1000 watts.

Nutrition Information

250 calories

6 g of fat

10 g of fiber

55 g of carbs

324 mg of sodium

9 g of protein

0 g of fat (saturated)

29 g of sugar

Ingredients

- Dandelion greens (1 c)
- Water (1 c)
- Spinach (1 c)
- Beet greens (1 c)
- Kale (1 c)
- Coconut oil (1 T)
- Green apple (1 cored)
- Stevia (1 tsp)

Kombucha, Cinnamon and Kale Smoothie

This recipe can be ready in 5 minutes, makes 1 serving (24 oz.), and will take approximately 45 seconds of blending assuming you are using a blender that is 1000 watts.

Nutrition Information

334 calories

10 g of fat (saturated)

35 g of carbs

18 g of sugar

22 g of fat

10 g of fiber

3 g of protein

187 mg of sodium

<u>Ingredients</u>

- Kale (1 c)
- Coconut oil (.5 T)
- Kombucha (1 c)
- Frozen papaya (.5 c)
- Cinnamon (.5 tsp)
- Spinach (1 c)
- Honey (.5 T)
- Flax seed (1 T)
- Ginger (2 tsp)

Conclusion

Thank for making it through to the end of *Smoothies: Healthy Green Smoothie 30 Day Plan to Lose Weight, Detoxify, Fight Disease, and Live Long*, let's hope it was informative and able to provide you with all of the tools you need to achieve your goals whatever it is that they may be. Just because you've finished this book doesn't mean there is nothing left to learn on the topic, expanding your horizons is the only way to find the mastery you seek.

One of the most important things to keep in mind while moving forward is that if you slip and eat something outside the scope of the 30-day plan it isn't the end of the world. Neither should you beat yourself up over your indiscretion unless you use your one mistake as an excuse to go completely off book for several meals or more. Instead, it is much more beneficial to remind yourself of all of the good work that you have done already and to get back on track as quickly as possible. Remember, detoxing and losing weight in a healthy and effective way is a marathon, not a sprint, slow and steady wins the race.

Furthermore, you are going to want to keep in mind that while you are likely to experience an increase in weight loss as your body adjusts to your new diet, it is only natural that this process will curtail itself as time goes on. Losing 1 pound of body fat per week is the average and more than that for too long of time isn't just unrealistic, it is unhealthy no matter what diet you are following. Focus on the physical and mental benefits that are sure to appear as you detoxify your system and let the weight loss take care of itself.

Finally, if you found this book useful in anyway, a review on Amazon is always appreciated!

Description

When it comes to easily getting all the nutrients that you need for the day while at the same time losing weight and detoxifying your system, there are few better options available than a green smoothie. While the idea of the green smoothie is relatively straight forward, any smoothie that is composed of at least 70 percent leafy, dark greens can be said to be green, the space is vast enough that it can be confusing for those just starting out to know where to begin. While the specifics might vary, all green smoothies are sure to share a variety of health benefits, regardless of the specific fruits and vegetables that you choose to use.

If you are short on time during the day but are still anxious to get your daily dose of nutritious fruits and vegetables, while at the same time losing weight and feeling better than you have in years then *Smoothies: Healthy Green Smoothie 30 Day Plan to Lose Weight, Detoxify, Fight Disease, and Live Long* is the book that you have been waiting for. Not only will you find 60 different green smoothie recipes, you will also get a meal plan that can be followed for a full 30 days to ensure that your weight loss and detoxification process is as simple and painless as possible.

Inside you will find delicious smoothies and recipes including

- Kombucha and Spinach Smoothie
- Dandelion Greens and Mixed Berry Smoothie
- Rolled Oats Breakfast Smoothie
- Agave, Spinach and Kale Smoothie
- Basil and Chlorella Smoothie
- Cayenne and Arugula Smoothie
- Tomato Pesto and Eggs Florentine
- Huevoes Rancheros with a Spicy Kick
- Butternut Squash and Lentil Soup
- Kale and Spinach Feta Wrap
- Tikka Masala
- Pasta Topped with Spinach and Homemade Tomato Sauce
- Cranberry Scones
- Carrot Cake Muffins
- *And more...*

www.ingramcontent.com/pod-product-compliance
Lightning Source LLC
Chambersburg PA
CBHW071156280526
45787CB00002B/525